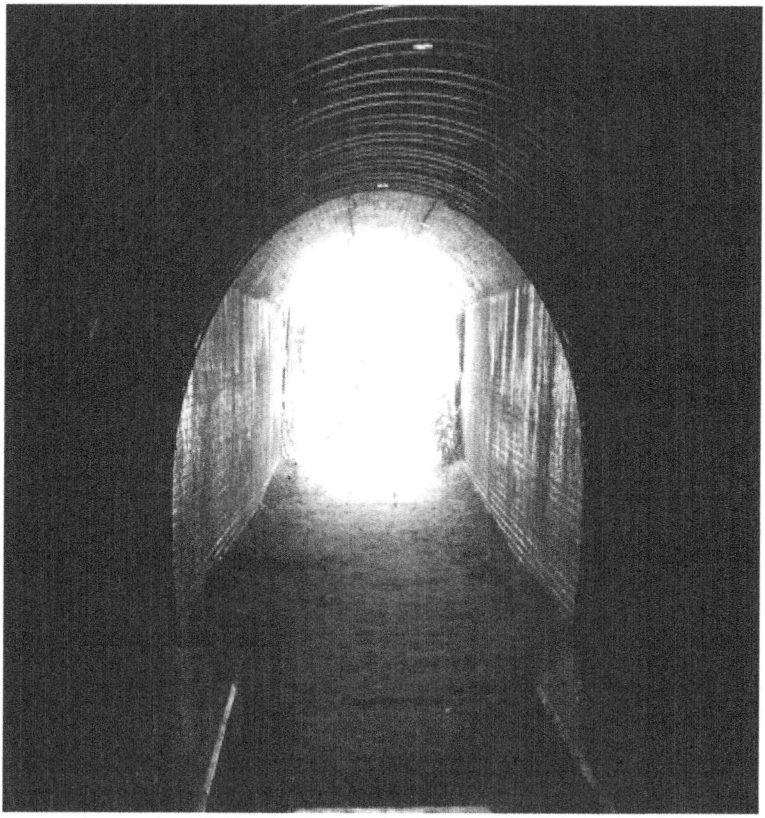

The Nightmare's Over

I Can Finally See The Light At The End Of The Tunnel

By Nancy Brown

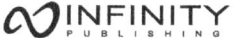

Copyright © 2011 by Nancy Brown

ISBN 978-0-7414-6678-5

Printed in the United States of America

Published September 2011

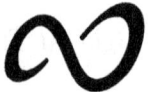

INFINITY PUBLISHING
1094 New DeHaven Street, Suite 100
West Conshohocken, PA 19428-2713
Toll-free (877) BUY BOOK
Local Phone (610) 941-9999
Fax (610) 941-9959
Info@buybooksontheweb.com
www.buybooksontheweb.com

TABLE OF CONTENTS

DEDICATIONS

To Doctor George Canallos, Doctor Eric Rubin, Doctor Rob Souffer, Doctor Jerry Ritz, Doctor Ken Anderson and Nurse Kathy Lynch, our thanks, love, and deep gratitude. Our gratitude extends to all the doctors, nurses, social workers, blood lab technicians and the entire staff of the Dana Farber Cancer Institute. Thank you to all the wonderful people at the former National Cash Register Corporation (NCR Corporation). We pray that God blesses you. Special thanks to Bob McKetchine and the 400+ people who came to give blood and platelets in Howard's name and honor. Special blessings to the dedicated few that still do.

__To our dearest son, Howard,__ thank you for always believing you would be here today. We are so proud of you. You never gave up and neither did we. We kept faith in you, our family and God and love kept us going through it all.
We love you,
Mom and Dad

__To our darling daughter, Cheryl,__ thank you for your unselfishness in saving your brother's life. You gave the most anyone could give in order to save his life – your bone marrow.
The love this family has for you is everlasting.
We love you. Love and kisses,
Mom and Dad

__To my husband, Marshall,__ thank you for your love and support for 44 years of marriage. You are my rock who helped keep us together as a family during this most challenging time. We have made a wonderful life together that I cherish every day.
I love you,
Nancy

__To my father, Mike Shapiro,__ who passed away November 28, 1992.
I miss you and love you always.

__To my mother, Lillian Shapiro,__ who passed away December 23, 2008, thank you for all your hard work in typing and writing this book with me. I know it was hard for you to remember this difficult time in your grandson's life. I love you and miss you.

__To my sister, Roberta Sufrin,__ who gives me unconditional love and support.

__To my sister-in-law, Carole Burnham,__ who gave me love and support.

__To my niece, Michelle Sufrin,__ thank you for helping with this book. I love you.

INTRODUCTION

Today, I am a 63-year-old wife and mother of twins, a woman and man, ages 43 years old. I cared for my family and worked for many years as an administrative assistant and receptionist.

In 1965, I was 19 years old, married and pregnant. It was not until my sixth month that I learned I was having twins – in 1965 ultrasounds did not exist. Marshall and I had mixed emotions. We were a young couple and had just moved from Worcester, Massachusetts to St Louis, Missouri for Marshall's new job with a large shoe company head-quartered there. I was excited and overwhelmed at the same time. My dream of motherhood was coming true. But, twins! I had no family or friends as support in Missouri.

Howard Scott and Cheryl Joy Brown made their entrance on March 10, 1966 in St. Louis, Missouri. Cheryl delivered at 2:00 p.m. and weighed 3 pounds, 7 ½ ounces. Howard delivered at 2:05 p.m. and weighed 3 pounds, 14 1/2 ounces. They were one month premature, beautiful and healthy. Twenty fingers, twenty toes.

Delivering a healthy baby is the universal mantra of all parents. My husband and I prayed for healthy children and on March 10, 1966 our dreams came true.

We took Howard home from the hospital first. He was a fighter from day one. Cheryl remained in the hospital for a few weeks in an incubator. It was heartbreaking to take one child home and leave your other child in the hospital. As soon as they both were home, the adventure began.

From birth, Howard and Cheryl had different personalities. They had different sleeping and eating habits. While Howard and Cheryl were newborns, we were in survival mode. My husband worked three jobs to support us.

It was difficult, but we managed through the ups and downs of the first year. Marshall and I were a team.

On May 24, 2010 I called my 44 year-old son, Howard, to wish him a happy 20th bone marrow birthday. He is in remission from stage IV T-cell Non-Hodgkin's Lymphoma, an aggressive blood cancer of his lymphatic system. I call it being "reborn" when on May 24, 1990 he started a new life. Howard's journey through the diagnosis, treatment and healing of his cancer reminds me of my two lives; life before his illness and life after the diagnosis. The day I learned my son had Non-Hodgkin's Lymphoma, the life that I knew shattered like a rock smashing a mirror. I will never look at life the same way again.

This is a story about my son, Howard Scott Brown. I share my sorrow and frustration when cancer ravaged my son and the joy of his recovery. Although this happened 20 years ago and medical technology has since improved and awareness of cancer has increased, my emotions and experiences as a mother dealing with the challenges of a sick child transcend time. I hope this account encourages other parents who face such a journey.

PART I – Howard

In 1984, Howard was elected vice president of his senior class at Framingham South High School. He was always outgoing, played basketball and had a great group of friends. He graduated from Babson College in Wellesley, Massachusetts, in December of 1987 and started his career as a Sales Account Executive in the Financial Data Processing Division of National Cash Register Corporation (NCR). Howard looked so handsome - almost six feet tall and fit at 180 pounds - in September of 1989 when he moved to Dayton, Ohio to take a new position as National Sales Manager in the Disaster Recovery Products Division at NCR's world headquarters. His new position meant traveling throughout the United States and Canada.

Howard's accomplishments made Marshall and me proud. As we packed his boxes to ship to Ohio we reminisced about his years at college and how NCR recruited him as an intern during his summer vacation. On September 15 we waved good-bye as he drove away. It was bittersweet. We were sad that he was moving far away from our home near Boston, yet we were happy about his new job and exciting career ahead.

Howard called that night from West Virginia and said everything was fine. He planned on arriving in Dayton Ohio, on September 18 and would check in at the Residence Inn until he found an apartment. Howard always put great effort into whatever he did, so it wasn't a surprise when he worked 15-hour days and enjoyed it.

A few days into his new job he called home. When Marshall answered the phone Howard sounded anxious, which was unusual from his pleasant, easygoing personality. He told his dad that he needed to talk to both of us. He said he had a large bump on his left upper cheekbone, near his ear, next to his left eye. Our first reaction was a bug bite or a pimple. Without cell phone cameras or Skype, which were still undeveloped, we were blind. We suggested he use a hot compress on the bump. He agreed to our suggestions so we decided not to worry. Little did we know our troubles were just beginning.

Fall 1989

On September 21st I took a few days off from work, packed and went to Ohio so I could help Howard set up his new apartment. Marshall drove me to Logan Airport for a 9:00 p.m. flight. I arrived in Dayton at midnight. When Howard picked me up I struggled to hide my reaction to a large red, black, blue, and purplish lump on the side of his face. Since we did not know any doctors in Dayton we decided we would both return to Boston to see our own family doctor. We set up his apartment with furniture, linens, dishes and the essentials and made plans to return to Boston. I left on September 24. Because of work commitments, Howard planned to follow a few days later.

Howard arrived on a Sunday. The lump had grown to the size of a golf ball. It prevented him from wearing his glasses. Marshall immediately took him to the Leonard Morse Hospital emergency ward in Natick, Massachusetts. The doctor on call examined him and declared it to be a cyst. He prescribed erythromycin and sent him home.

Howard had a bad reaction to the pills so on Monday morning, October 1, we called the doctor only to find that it was his day off. We were persistent in getting more information. We spoke with Dr. Stephen Frager who was the on-call doctor. When he heard Howard's symptoms he said to come over right away. On his examination he ordered an immediate biopsy. After the biopsy, Dr. Frager returned and asked Howard to come back to the operating room to have a second biopsy to send to another laboratory. I was at work and could hardly contain myself waiting for the report about

2

the terrible growth on Howard's face. I couldn't wait to go home. I needed to be with my family. I felt helpless waiting for information. I belonged with my son. I could not concentrate and thought I may have to quit my job if Howard needed more testing.

When I saw Howard and Marshall later, they said Dr. Frager felt Howard needed more tests. Howard's business itinerary was full and so on October 4 he left to speak at a seminar for the Massachusetts Chapter of the American Bankers Association. When he returned we went back to the hospital. At first Dr. Frager thought the growth was a cyst. When he drained it and examined it further he said it was not a cyst. He did another biopsy and stitched up Howard's cheekbone.

Before Howard left to travel to Philadelphia and then down to Tampa, Florida for business meetings, Marshall and I were frantic trying to figure out what the lump was imbedded in Howard's cheekbone. When he returned from his business travels, I took off from work to take Howard to doctors visits and endless tests at Leonard Morse Hospital in Natick, Massachusetts. They took many x-rays, blood work and vital signs. My company that I worked for as an office manager was sympathetic; I missed a lot of work. I had to put my son and family first.

We lived at the hospital for ten days straight. Not knowing was unbearable. I was irritable, nervous and lost 10 pounds during that time. The doctors and labs could not determine the diagnosis.

We struggled to stay positive, but it was agony waiting for test results to give us more information about Howard's condition. All the while, we did not tell many friends or family members because we did not want them to worry. Those were long days and endless nights waiting for telephone calls from doctors. Other than doctor's appointments, I was afraid to leave the house for fear of missing a call from the hospital. Weekends were the worst because the testing labs were closed.

I seethed at the idea of a closed lab while my family waited. It went like this - we expected a call on Friday. It never came. We called the lab at 4:00 p.m. on Friday and they told us the lab closed and to call the doctor on Monday for results. The time crept by.

Cheryl called constantly for updates. She lived with her college roommate about 15 minutes away from our home and worked full-time. I downplayed my frustration to lessen her worry.

On October 13, Howard had a CAT scan. They found that he was allergic to the contrast. Contrast is a dye doctors inject in a body to see everything in the Cat scan. Then Dr. Frager introduced us to Dr. John Jao, a tumor specialist and oncologist. Dr. Jao conferred with Dr. Frager and recommended Howard visit Dana Farber Cancer Institute in Boston, Massachusetts. They set up an appointment for us.

The morning of October 16 we left Framingham, stopped at Leonard Morse Hospital to pick up x-rays and medical results, and drove to Dana Farber Cancer Institute in Boston, Massachusetts. We arrived at 1:30 p.m. The waiting room was full. As I sat waiting I wondered what was wrong with each person. I wondered were they getting better. What stage cancer did they have? I prayed it was a mistake. Please don't let my baby be sick. I would gladly take his pain. My heart broke watching the children with cancer. It seemed senseless and unfair. Not knowing scared us. Our family felt alone in a waiting room full of sick people with cancer.

First a nurse directed us to fill out more forms. Then we met the head of the Oncology Department, Dr. George Canallos. He told us that Dr. Eric Rubin was going to handle Howard's case and would be his oncologist. Right away Howard liked him and put his full trust in him. He checked Howard from head to toe--a complete physical-- and then met with us to discuss the tests and reports. He explained that it was necessary to take more blood tests. He did another biopsy, plus a gallium injection with photos using nuclear medicine. He also did a bone marrow pull and aspiration so he could figure out what was going on in Howard's body. He explained that in doing a bone marrow pull they inserted a long needle and removed clear liquid from the bone marrow. It was an emotionally exhausting day, but we would finally get an answer.

PART II – The Diagnosis

It was not the answer we wanted to hear; "your son has cancer." They said Howard had Non-Hodgkin's Lymphoma, an aggressive blood cancer. We cried and hundreds of emotions ran through our heads. I held my baby in my arms and said we would get through this together. Drs. Cannellos and Rubin told us more tests were needed and they wanted to start immediately treating Howard with aggressive chemotherapy.

With heavy hearts we returned home and Howard left for New York on business. It seems crazy that after hearing his diagnosis Howard still wanted to fulfill his work commitments. We were all in shock and thought maybe he should live his life and work would be a distraction from the unbelievable news. Since he did not feel sick, he went to New York. He returned on October 19 and started in with the necessary tests that were ordered.

On that day his vital signs were high. The next day Howard endured another bone marrow pull and more blood work. Again, we waited for the results. Dr. Rubin told us the tests confirmed that Howard had Non-Hodgkin's Lymphoma (acute T cells), which is a disease of the Lymph Nodes. The Non-Hodgkin Lymphomas (NHL) is a diverse group of blood cancers that include any lymphoma except Hodgkin's Lymphomas. Types of NHL vary significantly in their severity, from indolent to very aggressive. Lymphomas are types of cancer derived from lymphocytes, a type of white blood cells. They are treated with combinations of chemotherapy, monoclonal antibodies, immunotherapy, and radiation. I learned there were 53,900 annual cases in 1989.

When they told us this we cried because we could not understand the finality of this disease when they said

Howard could die. No mother is ever prepared to hear that about her child.

Dr. Rubin explained the cancer was fast growing. There was no clear promise of a recovery, but the Dana Farber doctors and staff would treat the disease with aggressive chemotherapy, Howard, Marshall and I were three people in a car, alone with their thoughts and nobody uttered a word all the way home from Boston. Disbelief and shock overtook us. How could a healthy athletic young man be so sick that he could die? We did not understand. We were so afraid. It was a long ride home.

Chemotherapy appointments started the next week. I blamed myself because I smoked cigarettes. Was it my fault? Where else did I go wrong? I am his mother. Mother's protect their children. Could I have prevented the pain that Howard was going to endure? I could not stop crying. That week he took another battery of tests, some the same as in Leonard Morse Hospital. Each hospital found it necessary to take tests.

We could not put off any longer telling Cheryl. She was devastated. Being a twin, they have a special relationship. She could not imagine her world without him. Since birth they have shared toys, friends, classes and birthdays. Cheryl and Howard were the "wonder twins". They called themselves that since they were five years old. Wonder twins were part of a television cartoon "Super friends" that they would watch on television every Saturday morning.

I was glad Cheryl lived a few towns away unexposed to the day- to-day trauma of watching Howard experience the pain and side effects caused by the cancer fighting medications. I chose to quit my job when learning of Howard's diagnosis. My only job now was to help my son stay alive. Dr. Rubin gave me a book explaining the different types of Non-Hodgkin's Lymphomas. I read the cells in the Lymph tissues can begin to grow abnormally and if untreated can spread to other organs. Lymphoma is a general term for cancers developed in the lymphatic system. The most common type is Non-Hodgkin's disease. All other lymphomas are grouped together and called Hodgkin's disease. The lymphatic system is part of the body's immune defense system. Its job is to help fight diseases and infection. The lymphatic system includes a network of thin tubes that branch, like blood vessels into tissues throughout the body. Lymphatic vessels carry lymph; a colorless, watery fluid that contains infection-fighting cells called lymphocytes. Along this network of vessels are small bean shaped organs called lymph nodes. Clusters of lymph nodes are found in the underarms, groin, neck, chest and stomach. Other parts of the lymphatic system are the spleen, thymus, tonsils and bone marrow. Lymphatic tissues are also found in other parts of the body including the intestines and skin.

Like all types of cancer, lymphomas are diseases of the bodies cells. Healthy cells will grow, divide and replace themselves in an orderly manner. This keeps the body in good repair.

In the Non-Hodgkin's Lymphomas, cells in the lymphatic system grow abnormally. They divide too rapidly and grow without any order or control. Too much tissue is formed and tumors begin to grow and spread to other organs. The most common symptoms of Non-Hodgkin's Lymphomas are a painless swelling in the lymph nodes in the neck, underarm or groin. Other symptoms may include fevers, night sweats, and tiredness, weight loss, itching and red patches on the skin. Sometimes there is nausea, vomiting or abdominal pain. As lymphomas progress the body is less able to fight infection. We read and studied each word without completely understanding its meaning.

The T-Cell Lymphoma prognosis: T-Cell lymphoma originates in the T-lymphocytes, a type of white blood cell. It is a form of Non-Hodgkin's lymphoma. The prognosis in 1989 was a projected maximum five year survival rate. Five years was not enough time, but at this point we decided to think positively and take one day at a time. We relied on prayer.

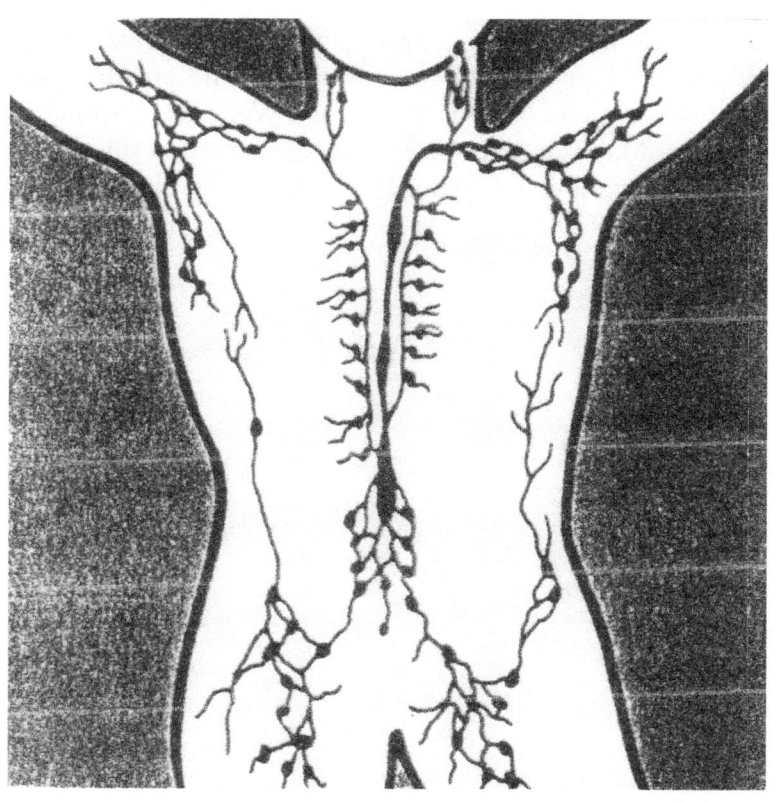

We discussed alternatives with Dr. Rubin. He said that Howard would need a heart scan and he would try a new protocol, M-Chop vs. Chope. On October 23, I became a full-time mom, nurse and driver - taking Howard for CAT SCANS, blood work and chemotherapy treatments.

Before Howard's first chemotherapy treatment my sister Roberta called to wish us luck and told us to inquire about a sperm bank. She told us the New England Sperm Bank and New England Cryogenic Center offer services to men. Those who would most often fill this category are: pre-chemotherapy and radiation patients, prevasectomy patients, oligospermic patients, occupational hazard and chemical workers, professional sports figures, absentee spouse and physically handicapped. Howard supported the idea to freeze his sperm so, if he lived, children were possible. I thanked her for this information because otherwise the chance of his having children in the future, would not be possible. We went to the sperm bank at the Newton Wellesley Hospital in Newton, Massachusetts. We learned years later that after being frozen for eleven years 75% of his sperm died.

PART III – The Journey

Fall 1989
Day 1, October 24

Howard signed a consent form and started his first round of chemotherapy at Dana Farber with a schedule where he would be an outpatient for the first three days. The treatments made him sick – he vomited and hiccupped constantly and developed a rash on his face. He was uncomfortable and his sleep was sporadic. This continued until the next round of chemotherapy three weeks later. Howard stayed in the hospital three days for this round.

The lymphoma spread to an ear, his neck and legs. These parts started to feel numb. For those three days I stayed in the hospital with him. Howard did not talk much. I could see he was doing much thinking. I asked questions, but he did not answer since he was in denial and depressed about his prognosis. My outgoing, talkative son stayed silent, which was not his personality at all.

I needed to keep myself busy so I started needlepoint projects to pass the long days and nights at the hospital and at home. The needlepoint I did was of an old yellow T-Bird car. To this day he has it hung in his office. I finished a needlepoint project every two weeks - mindless activity to keep my hands busy while I sat and watched my son go through hell.

October 26

After three treatments the lump that was growing on the side of Howard's head started to shrink. He had a terrible time trying to keep some food down, his skin broke out in rashes, vomiting and coughing gave him a sore throat and he lost 10 pounds He looked drained. His boss and friend, Mike

Brennan from NCR, took him to his home gym for light exercise. Although he was weak, he mentally wanted to go. He loved exercise and needed to feel that he had some control over his body. We were relieved that he had respite from the chemotherapy.

By October 31 he was continually in the hospital for chemotherapy and returned home after treatments. On a day that he felt a little better he went to the local Framingham, Massachusetts, NCR Corporation office for a few hours, made calls and caught up with work. He was grateful for the work; it gave him purpose. NCR was a blessing. All his hard work combined with his outstanding reputation as a salesperson played a role in why NCR was so compassionate during this trying time in his life.

Marshall and I decided to look only on the bright side and never show Howard any of our heartaches and tears. Howard has many friends and they rallied around him. He had his high school friends, college friends, work friends and neighbor's stopping by our house to cheer him up. They would reminisce about old times and talk about future good times they would share. We played Nintendo video games, board games, watched TV and read books together. We tried to keep his mind busy and distracted so he would not stay on his current pain and uncertain future. Cheryl came over the house often to keep Howard company. We sent word around to everyone that we would not tolerate any visits to Howard that were downbeat or accept any cards, letters or phone calls not on a happy note. We knew when Howard was upset or depressed and worked hard at keeping him entertained. Our main priority was his health. If small acts like having his friends come over to our house made him happy then we made it happen. But germs worried us because his resistance and immune system were low.

We made everybody who entered our home wear a face mask and rubber gloves. I cleaned my own house within an inch of its life. I needed to have control and make sure that cleanliness was to the highest standard. No dirt or dust anywhere. I could not rely on a cleaning service. We had too much at stake. I became a fanatical cleaner. We sterilized everything that he would touch. Howard's body was so weak from chemotherapy and eventually radiation that he could not afford to get sick.

We were told he would lose his hair and the thought broke our hearts at the first notice when we saw some of his hair come out we started to inquire about wigs that he could wear. We bought a wig, but Howard never felt comfortable with it on. It was difficult seeing clumps of hair on his pillow and in the shower. Eventually he shaved his head and wore a baseball cap. He never wore the wig.

November did not go well. Many complications set in and he found sleeping difficult. Howard developed a rash and more clumps of hair fell out. His blood counts and platelets dropped and it was an effort for him to go out. He was on Prednisone, Haloperidol, Benedryl and Trilafon, medicines to help control the pain. His taste buds disappeared so everything tasted bland and he suffered with a cough and chest congestion.

Around Thanksgiving he was invited to speak at his five year high school class reunion. Howard was his high school class vice president so naturally he was a good choice. We were glad that he felt well enough that night to attend. Howard is a motivational speaker. He spoke from his heart that night. He returned home pleased as all of his old school friends made him feel great and responded to his speech "To live life to the fullest because you never know what tomorrow may bring" with great applause. Cheryl told us he received a standing ovation for his speech. She said the room roared with applause. Going to his high school reunion and connecting with old friends brought him much joy.

Winter 1989

On December 2 Howard had a gallium scan. Technicians inject gallium into the body and take an x-ray to reveal if the cancer is still there. *It was still there!*

Dr. Rubin said he would try another chemotherapy regime called Chope. It required Howard to be in the hospital for five days. We arranged so Marshall and I would be with Howard during the process. I arrived there each day at 10 a.m. and stayed until 6 p.m. Marshall went to work every day and then relieved me at night. Cheryl came a few nights to spend time with her brother and gave Marshall and me a break.

Marshall and I did not talk much. We just kept moving back and forth from home to the hospital, feeling exhausted and helpless. Every time we tried to talk I cried. We had to believe the next treatment would work.

Marshall's frustration intensified. If there is a problem, Marshall solves it or fixes it. He is direct. He could not fix this. Howard's cancer and treatment were out of his control. We stayed in prayer for our son's survival and health.

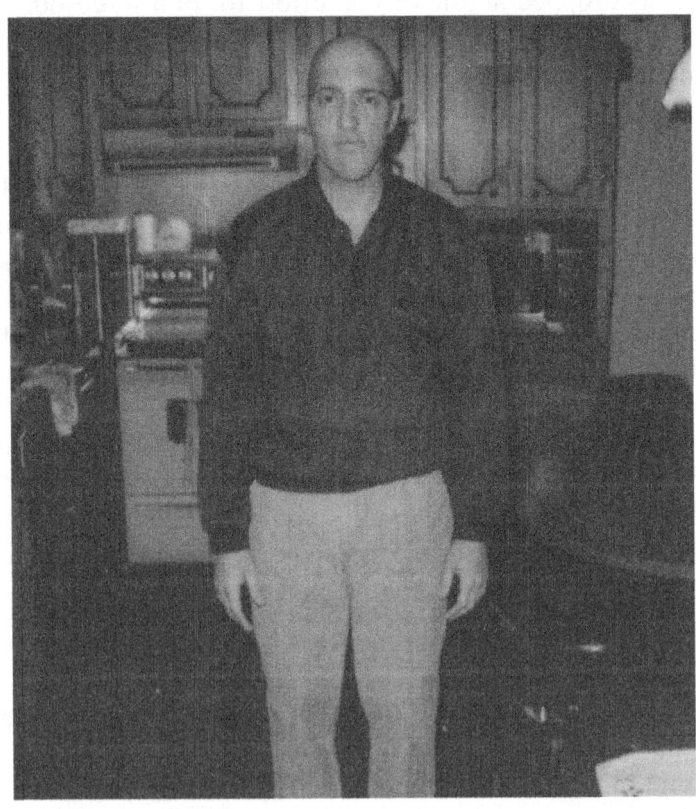

I stared at my sleeping son from the foot of his bed. Memories flickered through my brain - the day he first said "mama", his first steps, the day he learned how to ride his bike, the day he became a safety guard in fifth grade. I watched him in all the baseball, basketball and football games and when he got B'nai mitzvahed with Cheryl. I remembered his MVP award for high school baseball, his election as vice president of his high school class, his graduation from college a semester early, and now he was a successful business executive. I thought of all those moments, big and small, that made me proud to be his mother. Most of all, I thought of all the times he said he loved me. I could not imagine not hearing him say those words again. As he lie weak, thin and sick, I prayed for his health. I stayed with him in the hospital for five days and nights. *Our hearts broke! He could die.*

Winter 1989/1990

Howard came home November 20, 1989 he slept or just sat quietly in a chair, staring. It frightened us bad enough to call Dr. Rubin. Dr. Rubin explained it was not unusual for patients to react that way with the protocol Howard received. He said to expect Howard to be weak and tired. His chemotherapy and radiation and all the medication he was on had many physical side effects - headaches, body aches, dry mouth and rashes to name a few. The mental affects were just as difficult. There is no "normal" or "typical" with cancer. We constantly wondered if the protocols the doctors recommended were the ones that would save our son's life. No one knows what causes cancer; therefore there is no cure, only treatments to help Howard go into remission. Day after day, doctors put poison into his body to kill the cancer cells and day after day we wondered if this was the treatment that would work.

At the beginning of December, Howard's blood counts were very low. He finished that week with his first of over one hundred blood and platelet transfusions and I contributed three pints of platelets. On December 2 the oncology team gave Howard four days off from treatment to allow his body to recover.

Marshall and Howard flew to Ohio less than three months after he moved there to pack up his belongings. They put his furniture and car in storage for a while. Howard was placed on indefinite medical leave from NCR Corporation. Howard and Marshall flew home on December 5, only four months since Howard's promotion and the excitement of traveling throughout the United States and Canada. Marshall returned to Ohio again soon after to gather his belongings and put them in the car and drove back to Massachusetts and end his lease for his new apartment. Howard and Marshall did not talk too much about it. They just did what was needed. As a family, we decided that he could not be in limbo with part of his life in Ohio. He needed to be in Massachusetts, to continue going for treatment at Dana Farber Cancer Institute and focus on getting better. He wanted to focus on the present and do what was needed to get healthy. We thought positive thoughts. When he got well he could live anywhere in the world, even back in Ohio, if he wanted…when he got well.

After they returned from Ohio, Howard had to go in for another transfusion as his blood counts were low.

Every once in a while, when Howard was having a good day, he managed to get in two or three hours of work for NCR. He worked for them for four years. He originally started working for NCR as an intern from Babson College. He worked hard and was well-known throughout the organization. He was successful and a high achiever. He won many sales awards and recognition from top management at the company. They were so kind to him while he went through treatment. They continued to let him work when he felt well enough. The understanding and support that Howard received from NCR management was a blessing. The work was a diversion. It helped him focus on other things besides himself. It gave him purpose. He made an effort to attend the local NCR holiday party in Framingham and as Chanukah came about the same time he also attended a service at our Temple. Relatives and friends stayed connected with us daily. Every day that Howard could, he went with Marshall and I outside for walks. We talked about many subjects. On our walks, we spoke of stories from the past like family vacations. We chatted about present current events to focus on the world around us as a distraction from daily medical stats of white blood counts, red blood counts, and platelets. Marshall and Howard talked about sports. We discussed the future because we believed he would have a future. We talked about when he was better we would go on a family vacation to Disney World in Florida, just Marshall and I and Howard and Cheryl, like old times. I always tried to keep his spirits up.

At the beginning of January, 1990 Howard woke up and found new rashes on his body. We could not believe it. This whole ordeal felt like a roller coaster ride. We never knew what to expect. We called the doctor and Howard reported to the hospital for tests to determine what course of action to take. We tried to stay hopeful because we felt like we were in excellent hands and were getting the best care possible. A biopsy revealed the lymphoma again.

PART IV – The Transplant

A new protocol, E Sharp, went into effect with a higher dosage of chemotherapy. Five days of treatment left Howard with numbness plus toxicity and problems with his hearing. He suffered dizziness and night sweats, chills, headaches and exhaustion. He took sleeping pills, which helped a little. We could not understand why his body was not responding to the chemotherapy and radiation. Howard was out of choices.

We started discussions about bone marrow and transplantation, the last resort. In January 1990, bone marrow transplantation was experimental and a big risk. Once again, we had to be positive and thought that big risk would bring big returns. My son had to live.

First, Howard's immediate family was tested to find a match. We could be 0%, 25%, 50%, 75%, or 100%. We assumed Cheryl, being his twin, would naturally be 100% match, but that was not the case, being a fraternal twin, she had a 25% chance. If none of us were a match then we would have to hold a bone marrow drive and contact the National Bone Marrow Donor Registry for a match. Finding a match outside a sibling match is difficult.

He continued chemotherapy as we started the bone marrow process. He was continuing with his chemotherapy as an inpatient and was an outpatient for biopsies and blood work. He was taking the prednisone by injection and he grew weaker so he needed transfusions. His blood counts became dangerously low. He received antibiotics and more tests. Because of his condition doctors admitted him to Dana Farber. His temperature was 102.4 so his doctor Eric Rubin prescribed a red blood cell transfusion coupled with the antibiotics. Howard stayed at the hospital for ten days until his temperature came down and his nausea and diarrhea were under control. Marshall and I took turns being with him and walking him around the halls each day. His sister, Cheryl, was constantly with him helping to keep his spirits up. Finally he was able to come home.

When he came home, Howard was eager to go to Florida to see his grandparents. Dr. Rubin gave his permission but cautioned him to always wear a hat and use sunscreen protection. Howard felt it could be the last time he would see them. On January 20, 1990, we booked a flight to Florida to visit his grandparents, Rose and Leo Brown, who were not well enough to travel to Boston to visit. Howard's grandparents handled it well considering how different he looked since the last time they saw him - he had lost several pounds, had no hair and was weak and drawn. They were thrilled to see him and hugged him endlessly. We spent three days in Florida. When we returned we noticed hard purple lumps all over Howard's body and red blotches on his right arm, shoulders and head. He went back to Dana Farber for another biopsy that showed the lymphoma to be the same as before. This was a major setback. His protocol was the same as before called E Sharp. He went back into the hospital for intensive treatment for the next five days. This time he experienced loss of concentration, dizziness, rashes, numbness, intense nausea and his taste buds dulled. Watching Howard experience so much pain and misery killed me inside. I wished it was me. I wished I could trade places with him.

In February, 1990 Howard had a rash breakout with red dots on his neck and the back of his head. Dr. Rubin said it was from some of the medicine and recommended another type of chemotherapy. For the next three months he was given Methotrexate. It was an experimental chemotherapy. We went to Dana Farber weekly for an hour of treatment.

March 10 usually is a great day in our household since it was Howard and Cheryl's 24th birthday. Instead of a celebration Howard was having a Hickman tube inserted in his chest, because the veins in his arms could not handle any more needles. As we always tried hard to keep life as normal as possible, we reserved dinner for four at the Anthony's Pier 4 restaurant in Boston where we tried desperately to put on a happy face. It was a quiet dinner. I wondered what their next birthday would be like if Howard died.

After many different chemotherapy protocols and treatment, Howard was not getting any better. It was then the doctors decided it was necessary for him to have the bone marrow transplant. The doctor explained the procedure to us and gave us pamphlets. We let the word out that Howard was going to need a "match". We spread the word by telephone and emails. We would have shouted off the rooftops to bring people in for testing.

The NCR Company people arrived in droves to give blood samples. All of our immediate family came to help. His grandparents Lily and Mike came in from Worcester as well as my sister Roberta who flew in from New York. All Marshall's relatives came too including my sister-in-law Carole and brother-in-law Mark. Cheryl's friend Sue set up a blood drive at Dana Farber in which Cheryl's boyfriend Dave Gingras participated. Dr. Rubin explained that a mother was not a "match." However, if a match could not be found then, as a last resort, they would use my bone marrow. Again my heart broke. I wanted to be the match. Marshall could not offer his bone marrow as he remembered that twenty-three years ago he had developed hepatitis. Cheryl had a blood test to check her stats. While we initially assumed Cheryl would be a match because she is his twin, she had a 25% chance, the same as any other sibling. The bone marrow drive occurred between the time of Cheryl's test and when we received her results.

Two agonizing weeks. I believe that heaven smiled on us when the results showed Cheryl was a match, 10 for10. I didn't understand the numbers but it didn't matter, we were thrilled and excited and thankful to God for giving us twins. Perhaps that was the reason and God's plan.

Spring 1990

Dr. Rubin scheduled the bone marrow transplant procedure for the end of April or the beginning of May. Howard would continue chemotherapy protocol until then. In the interim the test of Howard's liver tested too high and he now had to wait for a couple of weeks until his liver function came back to normal. The wait was unbearable.

During the time we spent at Dana Farber Howard, Marshall and I made friends with other people who were also dealing with cancer. We met Marjorie, Candy, Richie, Christopher, and Mikey, who was only three years old. Slowly each one of them succumbed to this terrible disease while we were there. It hurt. There is something about being in the hospital and going through separate tragedies together. We got close to the other patients and parents in a short time. We understood one another. They touched our lives and we are better people for knowing them. Howard became especially close to a seventeen year old boy, Christian. They became fast friends while they were in the hospital and kept in touch after they each went home.

Dr. Rubin rescheduled Howard's procedure for May 24. We learned that since Howard would be in isolation before and after the transplant, there were several tasks to prepare him for the bone marrow. We sterilized everything which had to be germfree. We washed all of his clothing in hot water. After the clothes were put into the dryer and then, unfolded, put into a large plastic bag and delivered immediately to the hospital. We also brought a large calendar with a red marker so each day could be marked off, a new beginning of life for Howard. The calendar showed him that each passing day would bring him closer to leaving the hospital and on his road to recovery. We prayed the bone marrow transplant would work. With any medical procedure, there is no guarantee,

We arrived at Dana Farber on May 17 and were taken up to the 12th floor to room 1215, a room that he would spend three whole weeks in virtual isolation. The room had a bathroom, five shelves of medical supplies, a chair, bed and a small TV on which he could play his Nintendo and a refrigerator for medications.

On that day, Howard took a bath, put on his pajamas and at 5:00 p.m. readied for testing. Marshall and I went to dinner down the street. As the only outsiders allowed in Howard's room after the procedure, the nurse told us to return around 6:30 p.m. Howard's entire immune system would be wiped out. It was critical that he not get an infection, therefore, isolation. Even Cheryl could only look through a small window on the door. The nurse, Pat, told us we had strict procedures before entering his room. First, put a hospital gown over our clothes and tie it in the back. Second, wash our hands to be extremely clean. Third, put on a face mask. Last, put on rubber gloves. It was critical that Howard's room be germfree. His life depended on it. When we entered the room Howard became frightened since the procedure would wipe out his immune system. Doctors warned that it might not work. Both my children were undergoing medical procedures. We prayed a lot.

On Saturday, May 19, I arrived at the hospital early and watched Howard sleep as they had started the chemotherapy again, which would continue for two more days. Then on Monday I arrived at 7:00 a.m. and helped Howard prepare for his next step toward trying to stop the cancer from spreading - complete radiation. The nurses helped him into hospital pajamas, robe, slippers and a mask to cover his mouth and nose. They lifted him onto a gurney and covered him from neck to toes with a long sheet and his head with a towel to avoid contamination. All I could see were his eyes and I knew how scared he was. I was scared too. A nurse, a guard, Howard and I traveled by ambulance to Brigham and Women's Hospital across the street from Dana Farber. As we went through the corridor and then into an elevator they kept telling people ahead of us to turn their backs so no one breathed on Howard.

He received complete full body radiation twice a day for five days and then once on the last day. When he returned from the treatment he took a bath and got back into a clean bed. But he vomited constantly. The nurse gave him antinausea drugs trying to settle his stomach so he could sleep.

I spent each day with Howard and Marshall stayed all-night. We never left him alone, not for a minute. We needed to give him the security and love to help him through this horrendous ordeal. I held his hand and told him the bone marrow transplant would work. I did not eat or sleep much. The stress was unbearable.

May 24 finally arrived. After six months of treatment that had not killed the cancer cells, the day arrived. It was a sunny day and we took that as a good sign and were prepared for it. Marshall, Cheryl and I left our home at 5:30 a.m. to go to the Brigham and Women's Hospital. Cheryl had to be there for pre-operative tests and to give two pints of blood. At 8:00 a.m. doctors inserted a large needle 20 times in Cheryl's left hips and removed bone marrow. I stayed with Cheryl while Marshall was with Howard undergoing his last radiation treatment. It was difficult for me because I wanted to be with both my children at the same time. Cheryl's bone marrow extraction was at Brigham and Women's Hospital while Howard's transplant was at Dana Farber. It was only a quarter of a mile down the road, but it felt like a million miles away. Marshall and I talked often giving updates. While Cheryl had her operation, I sat in the waiting room and had great pain in my lower back almost as if they were doing the procedure on me. I felt my daughter's pain and could not stop crying. When Dr. Souffer came out of surgery he said that Cheryl was fine and her bone marrow was the best he had ever seen.

I hugged him and thanked him. I was so grateful. I told him that he held the lives of both my children in his hands. I ran down the hall and up the stairs and into a glass enclosed room and stood on a chair so Howard and Marshall would see me as they passed through the hall. The attendants stopped for a split second in front of the glass and I caught Howard's eye and put both my thumbs up to show him that everything so far was going great.

Meanwhile, the bone marrow was processed and sent over to Dana Farber for Howard. I went back to Cheryl's room and waited for her to come from the recovery room. Sitting alone in her room, I prayed for my children's health.

Marshall called on the phone and asked me to meet him outside the hospital on Francis Street. We arranged that he would now go to Cheryl and I would go to be with Howard. When I got to Howard's room I took him in my arms. He asked me to lie down with him and tell him a story. I knew how frightened he was of the unknown. My son was like a small boy again. It reminded me when I used to make up stories before bed when he was little. This time, as I lie beside my sick, weak son I told him happy stories of his childhood.

Later when I met Dr. Souffer he said that Cheryl had received only one pint of blood when she was supposed to have two. I was livid. I asked the nurses where the other pint of blood was and she said they neglected to order it. I told Marshall. He demanded the nurse get it now!

We were emotionally and physically drained. We had not slept or eaten in weeks. My son's life was in the balance determined by his body's acceptance of Cheryl's bone marrow. We could not let our guard down, even for a minute. Marshall and I had to be Cheryl and Howard's advocates. There was so much that was out of our control that we needed to control what we could.

Marshall and I met again in the street to make another change. I went to Cheryl and he went to Howard. I stayed with Cheryl until 8:30 p.m. when the staff asked me to leave. Cheryl was upset that I could not stay with her as it was her first time in a hospital. She was scared and worried about Howard. I kissed her good night and said that I would be back before she awoke in the morning. And I was.

24

May 24, 1990 was a long day and it wasn't over yet. I walked over to Dana Farber, "gowned" up and went into Howard's room at 9:30 p.m. Dr. Jerry Ritz, Dr. Christina Canning and Pat the nurse came into the room carrying a little bag, the size of an extra large tea bag. It was such a small amount. It looked like bubble gum. This little bag contained Cheryl's pink and white bone marrow. It was put into the I.V. bag and took only a few minutes to flow into Howard's body. This little bag of bone marrow could save Howard's life. We called Cheryl in her hospital room. Howard told her that he had received the bone marrow and it was flowing into his body. He told her he loved her and said "thank you for saving my life." Marshall and I and the nurses cried.

Howard stayed in the hospital for six weeks. Now that the bone marrow was in his body, he still had a 50% chance of rejecting it. Isolation started with the sweats, chills, headaches, nausea and jitters. Some of the day's events were so blurry and he had difficulty focusing.

Howard received constant attention. Nurses supplied many bags of platelets and blood, some still from donations made by Howard's friends, business associates and relatives. Being in isolation again meant that only Marshall, myself, and the nurses and doctors could be in the same room as Howard. Cheryl could still only see him through a small window on the door.

During the nights I sat and watched Howard sleep and during the days I watched him suffer. To pass the time I wrote letters to candy and video companies for donations to Dana Farber. We received 25 pounds of candy from one company. Another company sent 80 tapes of movies. The patients on the bone marrow floor were grateful for something else to do during their long hours of sleepless nights.

Howard did not eat for two weeks. His weight dropped to 135 pounds. He kept saying he was not hungry so the doctor brought in an I.V. which dripped for 12 hours at a time. Because of his low resistance, we were extremely careful about anyone approaching Howard that was not in perfect health - not even a sniffle.

Then, after 21 days, they opened the door of solitary confinement. No more antibiotics and Howard was moved to a new room. He was allowed visitors and Cheryl was the first. Both sets of his grandparents came to see him. Lily and Mike came. Rose and Leo traveled from Florida. He was thrilled. There was much love, joy and happiness surrounding Howard in the room that day. By Father's Day in June Howard was able to hold down some food and started to use his stationary bike in his room. He worked up to five miles on the bike and a couple of laps around the halls with his intravenous machine. Howard needed to listen to his body and not overextend himself, but he was determined and focused on going home.

PART V – The Homecoming

On June 20, 1990, Howard was discharged from Dana Farber. We took him home. He loved the big sign on the front of the house that read "Welcome Home Howard". We kept his return low key. Cheryl greeted us at the door and we had a quiet evening. My son was home at last and I felt relief. This was also the week of our 25th wedding anniversary and we gave thanks to God that our son was alive and home. Marshall and I did not want a big anniversary celebration. We were just so happy to be together as a family.

In July, Howard worked on building himself up by walking, and having a few friends over. During this time he developed pressure headaches and some canker sores. Sometimes he had neck stiffness and itching over his whole body, dizziness, coughs, and chills. We made many trips back to the doctors at Dana Farber. Howard's recovery was slow.

Although we expected some pain and discomfort, all through July there was not one day that went by that we were not upset by new symptoms, like the day he had chest pains and a severe headache. We rushed him to emergency room at Brigham and Women's for x-rays and blood work. He was given medication to ease the pain, and we returned home. In August, things got a little better. Occasionally he would have nausea, vomiting, heartburn and his hands swelled. He received regular checkups and blood work and Interleukin 2, an anticancer compound by a portable device that he wore on his belt.

Meanwhile, he was gaining weight. Every day he seemed a little stronger. I watched Howard carefully - I was his shadow. I kept him company all the time. I was so worried about a relapse.

Fall 1990

On September 27 we learned that Howard's friend Christian, the 17 year-old boy who he had met at Dana Farber, passed away. We were shocked and saddened.

Howard's weight was now 152 pounds and he needed to go to Dana Farber for his checkups for refills on his Interleukin pump cassette.

On September 29, which began Yom Kippur, Rabbi Splansky of our Temple invited Howard to take part in the services and prayers. Howard felt honored. He spoke about the fragility of life. It was beautiful and he made me so proud. Tears of joy rolled down my face. Now that Howard was home I found each day to be a holiday. He was starting to get well. We walked, we talked, and he slept and started to eat better. We cooked his food well done.

In October he attended the Stepping-Stones group which is a bone marrow survivor's support group. He thought it was wonderful as they all discussed feelings, families and even possible relapses. It pleased me that he was attending this group. These people understood exactly what Howard went through and continued to go through. They all had a connection. As much time as I spent with Howard, I did not have cancer nor go through the treatments. It was also a sounding board for him that was not his family.

In November 1990 Howard received a letter from NCR saying that he had won a trip to Hawaii. He had earned the trip from his sales success from right before his diagnosis. He was thrilled. He could not accept the trip then because of his illness. The company president offered it to him to use it even one year later. They were kind to him the last few years that he was ill and they said that when he was ready to go back to work they would offer him a position in California. He was now starting to feel a little better. His weight came back to 161 pounds and his vital signs were closer to normal. He started to feel more in control of his life. The bone marrow transplant was successful. Howard was officially in remission.

On November 19 we went down to Florida to spend Thanksgiving with Marshall's parents and to join them for their 50th wedding anniversary. Life had more meaning now. My son's life could have ended at age 24. We were celebrating love and life. Cheryl and Howard had a great time.

As we came into December and another year passed, we thought we could breathe a little easier. However, after the first of the year while away on business in South Florida, Howard experienced symptoms of chest pains with a cough and a cold, muscle soreness and tiredness. He made an appointment with Dr. Spiers at the H. Lee Moffat Cancer Center in Boston, Massachusetts. Dr. Spiers checked Howard thoroughly and determined that everything was good. Each time that I spoke with Howard I kept cautioning him not to work so hard and to rest more as his schedule was heavy, but it was difficult to hold him back.

In Early March Howard went to Hawaii, courtesy of NCR, and enjoyed himself with the 'old gang'. He returned home and attended a meeting of the Stepping Stones Organization. He spoke about relapse, work, drugs, relationships, family and friends. This is a wonderful organization that helped Howard cope with the stages of recovery. In April, he came back to see Dr. Sharon Bushnell, a plastic surgeon, to have surgery on the left side of his face on the ex-tumor spot that still showed faded lesions. Howard was feeling well. He wanted to have surgery to improve his face where the tumor first appeared. This was positive news and part of his recovery to move on.

On May 7 he flew into Boston from California for the operation. For the operation plus his regular physical checkup. A gallium scan showed face results were clean and complete; a bone marrow biopsy was also clean and negative; blood counts were at the lower end of normal but his kidney counts were high and normal. His weight was now 179 pounds. Dr. Rubin was pleased and directed Howard to eat right, get enough sleep and slow down.

On May 20, 1991 he moved to sunny California where he rented an apartment one block from the Pacific Ocean. His position for NCR Network Products was in Los Angeles. He chose to move to California for a fresh start. His new adventure far from home worried me as I prayed he would stay healthy. One day he discovered a few red spots on his body and immediately called Dr. Rubin in Boston who connected him with the UCLA hospital in Los Angeles. Medication relieved the symptoms. It pleased me that he was being careful.

In June, I went to California to help him set up his apartment. The last time I helped him set up his apartment in Ohio, he was diagnosed with cancer a few weeks later. He was doing well, his checkups were fine and he was feeling good and working 16 hours a day. He was back to his old self again. He met many new friends and spent time with them playing basketball and golfing. He also spent much time volunteering. He volunteered through the Big Brother Foundation and Jewish Federation. Howard felt lucky to be alive and gave back as much as he could through his time and his money to those less fortunate.

The next few years were good. Howard came home often to visit with us and to have his checkups at Dana Farber. Each year on May 24, the day of the bone marrow transplant, we celebrate and thank God that he is in remission for another year. It is a meaningful day in our family.

PART VI – Family First

In 1993 Howard became interested in the Jewish Federation, a charitable organization. During one of their get-togethers he met a lovely and charming young woman, Lisa, whom he fell in love with.

On September 3, 1993, another important day in Howard's life.-- He was an usher at his sister's wedding to David Gingras. Howard led the blessing over the wine and gave a toast. We danced all night.

In May 1994 Marshall and I gave Howard and Lisa an engagement party. We invited Howard's doctor from Dana Farber, Dr. Eric Rubin and his wife Kim. Howard presented Dr. Rubin with an award commenting about the care and dedication that he gave him. Guests cried during Howard's speech. Dr. Rubin was more than just Howard's doctor. Over the course of his treatment they became friends. No words can express how grateful we were for Dr. Rubin's expertise and care during Howard's illness.

On July 24, 1994 Howard and Lisa married in a traditional Jewish ceremony outdoors in California. One hundred and twenty family and friends traveled from across the country to celebrate Howard and Lisa's new life together. The foresight of freezing his sperm coupled with today's medical technology gave us a blessing that we are thankful for everyday - my smart, beautiful granddaughter, Emily.

Today Howard is the co-founder and CEO of a small internet social networking company. Since Howard owns his own company he can live and work anywhere in the United States. In 2005, Cheryl's husband, David got a job promotion to move from New York to Michigan. Cheryl and David and their three children, Marly, 7, and twins Danielle and Luke, 3, moved to Michigan. Since Howard's wife, Lisa, grew up in Michigan and her family still lived there, Howard and Lisa decided to move from California to Michigan so Emily could grow up with her cousins. In 2005, Howard, Lisa and their daughter Emily, 4, also moved to Michigan. Emily's two other cousins also live near her.

Today, Howard and Cheryl live 40 minutes apart. They celebrate holidays together. They attend their nieces and nephews soccer games together. They meet for dinner, just because they can. They experience everyday events that they could never do when Howard lived in California and Cheryl lived in New York. Emily is close to her cousins. They are growing up together.

We have a family tradition that we spend one week every summer in July in Ogunquit, Maine with relatives from Marshall's side of the family. We have been going for over ten years and the tradition continues today. To celebrate Howard's being in remission for 20 years, Marshall and I took our children and their families on a Disney Cruise in November 2010. It was a magical, joyful trip.

This is a true story from a mother's point of view. Although Howard has been in remission for 20 years, I shared my experiences, challenges, frustrations and joy in this book. My feelings are genuine and real. Howard kept a journal through his ordeal. The journal was an integral part of this book. Since Howard's cancer, my family is closer than ever. Tragedy can either tear families apart or bring them closer together. It brought us closer together. I am so proud of my children. Every day I count my blessings. Family first.

Love your mother, June, 2010

EPILOGUE

My daughter wrote this letter to Oprah Winfrey for a Mother's Day episode titled "Great Moms Getaway," which honored mothers. The letter was a surprise. It feels good to know that my children have always appreciated me.

March 10, 1999
Great Moms Getaway
P.O. Box 811071
Chicago, IL 60681

Dear Oprah,

When I was younger I was a well-behaved little girl. But like any child I had my moments. During those times my mother used to say, "wait until you have children of your own, I hope they act just like you." That day has come. Six months ago, I gave birth to a baby girl. Becoming a mother has given me a new perspective and I have a greater appreciation for my mother. Suddenly, it is not about me anymore. Mothering is the most selfless, giving and rewarding job in the world.

Growing up my parents stressed how important a positive attitude was. My mother is an upbeat, vibrant woman. Her positive attitude is contagious. That became especially meaningful when my twin brother was diagnosed with cancer. At the age of 24, my brother was not only losing his hair and losing weight from the chemotherapy and radiation treatment but was at risk of losing his life.

My mother dedicated all her time, energy and efforts to care not only for my brother, but also for the other patients at the Dana Farber Cancer Institute in Boston, Massachusetts. My mother walked through the hospital with a smile on her face. She would tell stories. I remember her telling the story of when Howard and I were 3 years old we had locked her out of the house. She was pleading with us to let her in, but we just giggled. We would not open the door, eventually, she had to get a ladder and climb through the window into the kitchen sink. She made others laugh for a brief moment so they could forget about their pain for awhile. She would even bring the nurses little gifts to recognize their hard work and to show her appreciation.

My brother's cancer left my family feeling helpless. Instead of dwelling on the situation, my mother channeled her energy into positive activities. She organized a blood and platelet drives at the hospital. She contacted friends, acquaintances, relatives, neighbors and co-workers. Four hundred people showed up to offer their support. This act of kindness benefited many people in need of blood and platelets. In addition, she wrote letters to candy and video companies for donations to the Jimmy Fund. A number of companies responded to my mother's letters. One company sent 25 pounds of candy to the hospital and video stores mailed in over 80 videotapes for patients to watch while receiving treatment.

Being a twin I was 100% bone marrow match for my brother. In May, it will be 9 years since the bone marrow transplant and fortunately, my brother is healthy, successful and happily married. I honestly believe that along with medical technology, his positive attitude played a key role in his ability to survive.

That is one of the attributes that both my brother and I have learned from my mother. My mother is a kind, generous, honest, caring person and a terrific role model. I

admire her and look up to her. I hope that one day my
daughter will describe me exactly the same way.

In the meantime, I know it would mean the world to her
to be recognized by the Oprah show for the one thing that
always been foremost to her: being a wonderful mother.

Sincerely,
Cheryl Brown

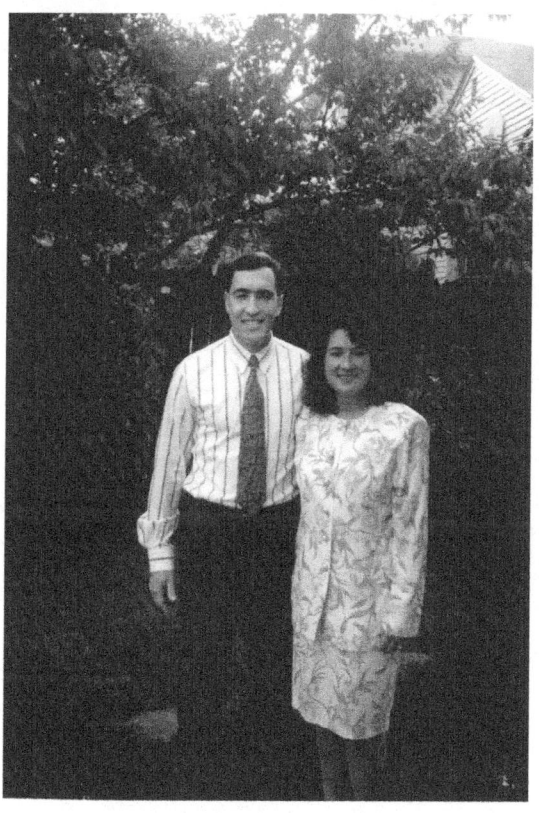

Wonder twins September 1993

Made in the USA
Monee, IL
07 July 2026

56551269R00030